MACROBIOTIC

CHILD CARE

CORNELLIA AIHARA

First Edition   1971
Revised Edition
    1st printing   1979
    3rd printing   1984

The George Ohsawa Macrobiotic Foundation is a non-profit public membership organization whose purpose is to make macrobiotic information available to the public.

To this end it publishes the works of the late George Ohsawa, the founder of the modern day movement, and those of his students Herman and Cornellia Aihara. Other macrobiotic books are also distributed, and the Foundation's monthly magazine is sent to members.

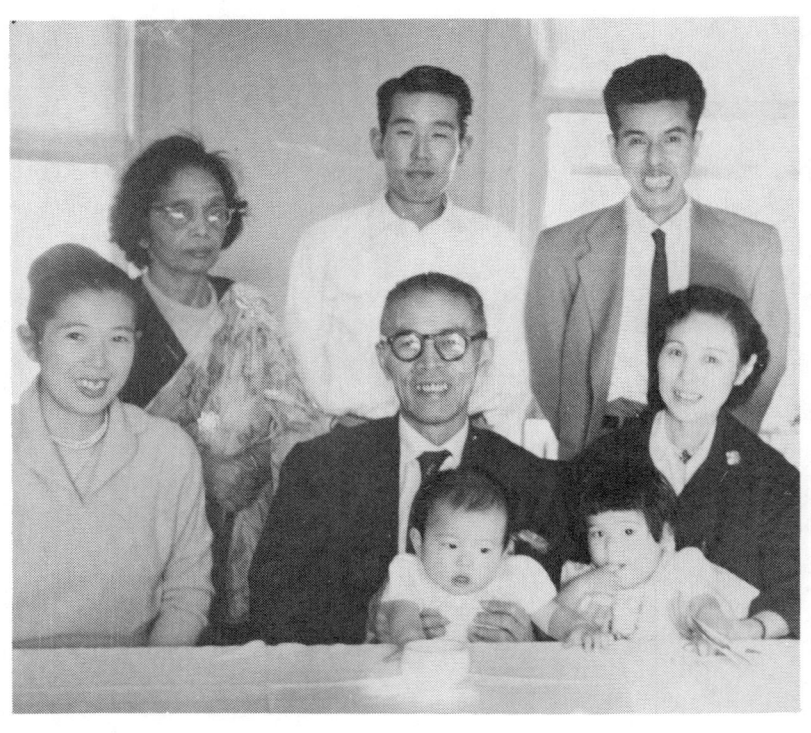

Dr. Shakuntara Rao   Tadahiro Yokota   Herman Aihara

Cornellia Aihara   George Ohsawa   Lima Ohsawa

                           Jiro Aihara   Marie Aihara

About the Author

Cornellia Aihara was born in Fukushima, Japan. She began macrobiotic study in Tokyo at the school of George Ohsawa, the founder of the modern movement, and was assigned as a sales girl to sell Ohsawa's weekly paper, *World Government*, on the streets of Tokyo. From this she says, "I learned the most important lesson of all; how to reduce exclusivity and what is real brotherhood — how to be a happy person." Being a newspaper sales girl, she missed the cooking lessons at Ohsawa's school, but she learned instead that which is the foundation of macrobiotic cooking and life — brotherhood without exclusivity.

She later came to the United States and married Herman Aihara, a leader and teacher of macrobiotics in the U.S., and the founder and president of the George Ohsawa Macrobiotic Foundation. Their daughter Marie was born in 1958, and their son Jiro was born in 1959.

Cornellia studied cooking with Mrs. Lima Ohsawa in the United States, assisting her in cooking at macrobiotic summer camps from 1960 to 1964. Since 1969, she has been passing along her knowledge of macrobiotic cooking, traveling with Mr. Aihara to communities in the United States and abroad.

From George and Lima Ohsawa she learned the philosophy of macrobiotic child care; from Marie and Jiro she learned its art and practice.

This book is an expression of her gratitude to her teachers, Mr. and Mrs. Ohsawa, and to all macrobiotic friends in Japan, Europe, and America.

cover art by Lori Pack

Contents

CHAPTER I

Child Care

Macrobiotic children seldom cry

Many babies and small children came with their parents to the Big Sur Summer Camp in 1969. I was very surprised that these children cried so much. At the 1960 and 1961 New York Summer Camps one mother brought her six-month-old baby. She helped Lima Ohsawa and me in the kitchen. Her husband came only on weekends. My daughter Marie was 2½ years old; my son Jiro was 1½ years old at that time, but I helped Lima prepare three meals a day for two months. In the morning someone else helped with the dishes but for lunch and dinner my friend and I had to do the dishes and pans by ourselves. On the weekends there were sometimes one hundred people. The children stayed in a cabin and I set aside one hour a day to play with them. Although I spent very little time with my children, they did not cry without reason. From that point I realized that macrobiotic children do not cry unnecessarily.

What did George Ohsawa have to say concerning the care of children? I remembered what George taught us and decided to write these articles.

Don't hold your baby too much

At the end of 1959 George Ohsawa came to America for the first time since World War II. George and Lima stayed in my home. One day George held Jiro for half the day. I said to

George, "You taught us not to hold our babies so much." He smiled and said to me, "Parents should not hold their baby, but I am the grandfather, so it is all right."

A mother's daily life is very busy, so only hold the baby to feed him or to change his diaper and then leave your baby alone in the crib in a quiet atmosphere. This is the start of your child's education. I learned this from George Ohsawa. When a baby cries between feedings, just change his diaper— do not keep holding him. If you are too solicitous to your baby, he thinks he has control over you.

The mother should set up a schedule for feeding her baby. In this way she knows whether the baby is crying from hunger or a wet diaper. Sometimes he has a different cry— perhaps a diaper pin is sticking in him and causing pain. So take care of this. In Japan, sometimes a baby cries because of a stomach ache. Usually, the nursing mother is unable to eat raw dry soybeans because it has the taste of green grass. However, if the soybeans taste good to the mother, then she knows her baby is crying from a stomach ache.

When a baby cries and has a red face, the mother can tell if the baby has a fever by touching the baby's forehead with the tip of her tongue. If you have no thermometer, this is a quick method. Your tongue will feel hot if your child has a fever.

When parents do not hold them so much, children become more open to other people. If guests come to visit, the children open their arms and welcome being held. First-time guests always enjoy this warmth. These children are never shy because they are not overly attached to their parents.

When Marie was five months old she caught the German measles. Her face was red from the fever. I held Marie in my arms by our back door overlooking our yard. This was the first time I held her for a long time, so she smiled at me with her red face. Non-macrobiotic children usually cry when they are so seriously ill. Being very sentimental, I cried inside watching Marie smiling. I appreciate George Ohsawa's teachings. As a child I was very sickly and always caught colds and had heart trouble also. I kicked off my covers continually and my mother didn't know how to take care of me. Although I didn't cry, I was very uncomfortable and often moaned and sighed. Remembering this, I can see how Marie's infancy and mine were so different.

The spirit to produce breast milk

One time when I was breast feeding my baby, Lima-san brought a letter into my room. She said that at feeding time it is not good to have an empty mind. I should read a book, study and try to educate myself more. George Ohsawa was always concerned with saving time. A busy mother seldom has time for outside reading. I never followed this advice because I liked talking to my babies when I fed them. Now, however, I understand and appreciate this teaching.

Two months after Marie's birth, I took a cool bath and caught a cold. Having no appetite for three weeks, I just drank water only. My dream was to give my baby my own milk. So I was able to produce milk from water alone, but I lost thirty pounds. At birth my heart had an extra Botalis pipe. In my childhood I had heart trouble, so doctors and fortune-tellers told me I would die by the time I was 19 years old. But even though my health was bad I could still produce milk by my will. Macrobiotic food is most important in producing good quality breast milk, but it is also important for the mother to have a deep faith and a strong desire to produce high quality milk for her baby. I was not healthy, so this will was necessary. When a mother gives milk to her baby, only she knows the peace and happiness of breast feeding her baby.

Food to produce breast milk

During pregnancy a mother's food is very important; after birth this is also true. I breast fed Marie for two months, Jiro for about thirteen months, and had no trouble. You realize that taking care of macrobiotic babies is easy. They are not so much trouble, so give thanks for having a macrobiotic baby. After giving birth, every morning I ate two bowls of miso soup. At snacktime, I ate whole wheat noodles. If you have no appetite, it is because your body is tired. At that time I took hot cow's milk with yannoh (1 cup milk to 1 tablespoon yannoh). This is not so good, but to feed the cow's milk to the baby is worse. After taking this, breast milk is soon produced. Azuki bean rice with vegetable tempura is also good for producing a lot of breast milk. When I lost my appetite, I always ate azuki bean rice. If a mother has normal breast milk, she is hungry often.

Once, Jiro had a fever of 100° in the summer. At that time we lived in Manhattan close to a doctor. We called him. Herman thought I needed the comfort of a doctor. He said nothing was wrong, because Jiro had an appetite. I began to think—I wondered why Jiro had a fever. Three days before, we had gone out to a Chinese restaurant with a friend. I had some soup made with pork stock. The baby was sensitive to animal protein. After that, I never went to a restaurant until I had stopped breast feeding my babies. When you are pregnant you cannot see what food is doing to your baby, but when you are breast feeding you can see very soon the effect of food. After birth, the baby tells you if the food you eat is a good balance or not. Sometimes the taste of the food appeals to the mother, but the baby doesn't like it.

Mother learns only through experience

George Ohsawa said, "A mother must learn by herself to take care of her baby; you cannot teach her." If you want to have a good baby, then you must be a good mother. Every day children observe their parents' life, so it is not necessary to formally teach them. You can see that small children understand what their parents are doing from their daily life. After we moved to Chico, our house had a small yard. Our children were free to play there. They played with pie pans and kitchen utensils. George Ohsawa said not to give children toys, because this stops their imagination. Our neighbor's older children copied Jiro's ideas. I always smiled at their play. It was a part of their own idea. When Marie was four years old, a friend of mine took her to the Sacramento River. There, Marie collected stones. Our friend asked why. She answered that she would bring them home to mommy to make pickles. We laughed.

If you have a baby at home, you learn many things from your children's minds. When I had my last baby, Marie and Jiro asked me why I went to the hospital to have a baby. Tama, our cat, had five kittens at home. I was ashamed. I answered shamefacedly that my body was not healthy, so I had to go to the hospital. People who lived in former times were very hard working and had many children born in the fields or outside. Now many macrobiotic people do the same thing. I heard and am very grateful to them for using natural childbirth. In this country, some midwives recommend this method but most pregnant women go to the hospitals. But macrobiotic people are returning to old customs, so I am very thankful. Sometimes my children ask me why Tama, our cat, eats my food. Why doesn't she cook for herself. Children think that animals and humans are not different. They don't separate them; they think they are the same. They understand everything from oneness. Every child has this knowledge by birth, but I believe 'education' hinders this thinking from developing.

Food during pregnancy

Macrobiotic women usually do not have morning sickness. If they have morning sickness, then their food is not a balance of yin and yang. You must figure out for yourself this balance. In Japan, when a woman discovers that she is pregnant, she suddenly has a craving for salted plums. In the beginning, a woman needs more acid food. Lima said this is because the baby needs calcium. If she doesn't have enough calcium for her baby, then a woman eats salted plums. This takes the calcium from her teeth and gives it to the baby, who needs it. I didn't like salted plums, so I ate fresh sour plums in my early pregnancy. George Ohsawa said that if a mother eats simple food and works hard, it is very good for her baby.

Ear lobes

The ear lobes of a baby tell what kind of food the mother ate during pregnancy. A large ear lobe indicates the yin part of the food taken by the mother during pregnancy. If the baby's ears lie flat against his head, this indicates the mother worked hard and ate salt. In Japan, a woman cannot indulge her whims when she is pregnant because her husband's parents live with them. Lima told me that my daughter's ears were not so good, because I didn't have my husband's parents living with us. We did have two friends living with us, but I didn't have to be so reserved because of them. My friend says many American children have well-shaped ears and good lobes. She thinks this is because Americans eat fruit (yin) and meat (yang), so this balance produced good ears. If a baby boy has good ears and small eyes, this is a good sign, but big ears and large eyes are caused by fruit. What do you think? My friend and I were careful with fruit during pregnancy, so our children's ear lobes are not so big.

My pregnancy

When I was six months pregnant, Herman went to Miami. There he had trouble with the Immigration Department with his visa, so he couldn't return. At that time we owned two stores, Azuma and Yamato—Japanese gift shops. I took care of the Yamato store. Besides this I was taking classes in night school until ten o'clock. My home was in Long Island. The school was in Manhattan. Therefore, I had to take the subway home. Often I arrived home after midnight. Thus, I slept only four hours a night. Of course, I didn't have much time to spend cooking. My favorite food was ice cubes, because my body was so hot. Since I also took care of two brothers who were living with us, I prepared their food and took care of the store. So sometimes I also enjoyed ice cream. In the middle of December, Herman came back from Miami. Then a Japanese friend came to visit. When we took him to the train station to depart, it was a very cold night. However, I craved ice cream. I told this to Herman. He said since I was very active, if I wanted to eat ice cream, I should. I was very comfortable with what he said. I didn't eat fruit during my pregnancy, because once I began, I couldn't stop. Fruit was my favorite food. When I was nine months pregnant, I ate half a grapefruit, because I craved it. This relaxed my body. Then a few days later, labor pains began. I hadn't eaten meat for a long time, so fruit was very hard on my body. Before I married, when I menstruated sometimes there was pain. Then I recalled that I ate fruit during that month. Many people say pregnant women should eat a wider diet—not follow a strict macrobiotic diet. But pregnant women are not sick. It is better to eat regular daily food with gratitude and avoid any trouble. A little fruit is all right in season, but green vegetables or old pickles which are more acid from natural fermentation are better to eat. These are better than fruit. In Japan, they say purple-colored food such as eggplant, figs and grapes can easily cause a miscarriage. So the Japanese do not give these foods to pregnant women. Also, pregnant women should not eat persimmons because they cool the body. One friend of mine in Chico baked a persimmon cake when she was pregnant. George Ohsawa said to me that she shouldn't eat this cake, because it can cause a miscarriage.

Miso Soup

When I was living in Chico, five macrobiotic women got pregnant at the same time. Four women were a little anemic, so their doctor suggested iron pills for them. Of course, no one took them. If you are pregnant and anemic, you are eating too much fruit or drinking too much water. Eating too much other yin foods can also make you anemic. Decrease your salt intake. One woman was not anemic during pregnancy because she ate a bowl of miso soup every day. Perhaps due to the salt of the miso, she had a baby boy while the others had baby girls. If you strictly follow a macrobiotic diet of grains, vegetables, seaweeds and beans, then every day you need miso soup. Otherwise you will crave dairy products during your pregnancy, especially after the birth when you are breast feeding your child. While my friend and I were in the hospital for five days after giving birth, we had no miso soup there to eat. Our bodies craved dairy products, especially milk, so we drank it. When we returned home and were able to eat plenty of miso soup each day, we stopped craving dairy products. This is my experience. I think maybe milk and miso fulfill the same craving in our body. However, miso is better quality than milk. Miso is vegetable but it is more yang because of the salt. Miso soup cleans nicotine toxins from the body. It is not recommended for a mother to smoke during pregnancy. However, if you do smoke, you need miso soup every day to help protect your baby. If miso soup is too strong for you to eat, just use a little bit of miso to taste so the soup is like a clear broth.

Activity During Pregnancy

After the baby is born, it can bring happiness or sadness to your home depending on your food and how orderly your life was while pregnant. So, during pregnancy, a woman should maintain her daily routine the same as before pregnancy. If the body is always active, then the birth will be easy. If the mother has nothing to do, she becomes lazy. Then the baby grows fast—it becomes too big. In old Japan, a samurai lord's wife had nothing to do. However, when she was pregnant, she spread seven cups of soybeans in one room and picked these up while she was wearing four inch high wooden shoes. This daily exercise made her bend her body, so the baby didn't grow so fast. Also her hips became stronger, so the birth was easier for her.

If you are pregnant, do not take strong yin food and your baby will have a strong stomach. If the stomach is strong, then the child will not easily get sick, because all diseases begin with a weak stomach.

Bowel movement of the baby

When a mother begins to feed her baby cereals, his bowel movement becomes harder and longer. When the baby just eats his mother's milk, the bowel movement is softer. It is better for the bowel movement to be long and large. One day my children forgot to flush the toilet; Lima saw their stool. "How wonderful," she said, "a long, big stool, and just one. Even I can't have a bowel movement like this." So we have great gratitude to the macrobiotic diet for our healthy children. Do you watch your children's stool? When Jiro began to eat brown rice, I was washing his diapers in the toilet and noticed many grains from his stool floating on top of the water. I picked one out, because I was worried about his digestion, but it was only the skin of the rice; the inside was digested. Since the baby doesn't chew well, he cannot break down the skin. So don't worry if your baby doesn't chew well enough. If the stomach is strong, the grain will be digested.

When baby first walks

Breast fed babies normally walk at 14 to 18 months old. Babies fed with cow's milk usually walk before they are one year old. Cow's milk has more protein (yin) and calcium (yin), so their bodies grow faster (yin). In Japan, if a baby walks before his first birthday, they make mochi using 7 cups of sweet brown rice, put this in a sack and tie it on the baby. It is difficult for the baby to walk, because they have not developed their balance. This slows them down. To me this makes the baby more yang. Some macrobiotic children walk very slowly, but their teeth grow normally; don't worry, their bones have enough calcium. At age two the baby should be walking. My friend's baby boy was four years old before he began to walk. George Ohsawa said, "Walking later is better, the brain instead is growing. If a baby is too active walking, all his energy goes to his feet, not to his head." Lima said that four years is too late to begin walking. But George said that the later the better. Cow's milk makes a baby fat and healthy in appearance, but his judgment grows slower. For this reason mother's milk is better. For the development of the large brain, human's milk contains everything that the baby needs; cow's milk lacks this. So different milk produces different kinds of judgment. If you had no milk, would you give your baby the milk of a cat or dog? Americans don't look at it from this angle, because they have been accustomed to drinking cow's milk for such a long time. The Japanese would never substitute cow's milk for human, but would call a wet nurse. This woman was called the breast mother and the children she nursed were a breast family. How would you feel if a cow was part of your breast family? We never considered substituting cow's milk for mother's milk, because we did not want to be part of a cow's family. Another substitute for breast milk was rice milk. This is rice milk I, for a baby three months old or so, different from rice milk II, for infants:

> Soak brown rice overnight, grind it in a suribachi, then cook it soft with a lot of water. Add amasake or yinnie syrup to make it sweet, similar in taste to breast milk.

Bowed legs and other problems

Jiro's legs bent when he began to walk. I thought this was because his body was too heavy. Also I was pregnant every year for three years straight. Jiro was the last baby, so possibly he was weaker because of my condition. George Ohsawa said, "Only macrobiotics can make his legs strong. This is the normal way. Drugs cannot cure this." George told me to study how to cure this myself. Before Jiro began to walk, we went swimming at the ocean with George and Lima. Jiro ate lots of sand there. George said to me that Jiro lacked minerals and to feed him brown rice mixed with another grain.

At the New York summer camp, a four year old boy sucked his thumb all the time. George asked me whether my children sucked their thumb or not. I answered that I had enough breast milk so my children didn't need to suck their thumb. George said that if a child sucks his thumb, he lacks minerals. Later Jiro began to suck his thumb in school sometimes. He was older, so it seemed he did this because of a complex. So a mother must study why her child sucks his thumb. It is not normal. The cause can be a lack of minerals, lack of salt, or a complex.

After the New York summer camp, we traveled in Europe for six months, then we returned to New York City. There I began to feed Marie and Jiro the head and bones only of small fish. I split the head of the fish down the center, opened it flat, then floured it and deep fried until it was crisp. So before we moved to Chico, the children thought fish was only head and bones, no meat. A year and a half later, Jiro's legs straightened out. I am very grateful to the macrobiotic diet for this.

For her first pregnancy a woman has enough excess stored to give the baby all he needs to form a healthy body, but in her third pregnancy or later a woman may need carp soup in order to have a source of calcium to produce a strong baby. This depends on the mother's condition. Carp soup is a good balance—carp is a very yin fish and burdock is a yang vegetable. This is cooked for a long time (see *Koi-Koku*, **The Calendar Cookbook**).

If you eat a lot of mochi during your pregnancy, your baby will have much endurance when he grows up. When a mother makes mochi she puts a lot of love and care into it. She makes very yang mochi which are a good snack for the children. If your baby is skinny, feed him mochi; he will gain weight and his muscles will become stronger.

How to make your child strong

When I wrote this article I recalled many things George Ohsawa said. Remember, children are the mirror of their parents. When you observe a child, then you know what kind of parents he had. I emphasize this again—*don't hold your children too much*. Observe mother cats and mother dogs; they just feed their children and clean their bodies, then they go outside. Kittens and puppies are very quiet; they do not cry. So I told my children, "Look at the kitty. He still has his eyes closed, but when his mother leaves him, he doesn't cry. But you always cry when I go out." My children were ashamed when they realized this.

At the entrance to the New York summer camp in Southampton, there is a large forest with small cabins. The road is gravel. George Ohsawa saw Marie putting on her shoes. He told me to take them off. The feet are the most yang part of the body. If you keep them cold then the internal organs will be stronger and healthier. So I took off Marie's shoes and socks, but the small stones hurt her feet; she was very unhappy. The camp had one kitten named Sesame. I said to Marie, "Look at Sesame, she has no shoes, but she doesn't cry. Even though she is so tiny, a real baby, she wears no shoes." So Marie never complained after this.

In my New York home, there were wooden floors, but the children always went barefooted, even in winter. They began to catch cold sometimes—to sneeze and cough—so I put socks on their feet, but soon they would take them off. I also cut off the feet of their pajamas, so they could be barefooted. We do not like to sleep with socks. In Japan, some people sleep with their socks. They say these people can never meet their parents when they die, because they will die first. Babies are very yang, so they do not need many clothes and can go barefooted. This is a good custom to follow. In New York, the winter is very cold, but inside the house it is very hot. It is easy to ruin your child's health.

Taking the baby outside for a walk in cold weather is very

beneficial for the child's health. All people, even babies, should go outside in cold weather, but it is not good to take babies out when it is raining. A baby can go out when it is 1½ months old; before that a mother may still be weak. As your child grows, has no diseases and stays healthy, you understand and are very grateful for macrobiotics.

My history

I was a very weak child, so I am glad that my children are active and strong. My friends say to me that they don't believe in macrobiotics because I'm not strong. I know my health is weak, but others do not realize my past condition. My family doctor told me I couldn't get married. Now I have two children and the doctor is very surprised to hear this from my mother.

Modern doctors in New York told me that my veins were getting smaller and that I could die any time. They wanted me to have still another heart operation, but I refused. I was born with an abnormal heart. That I am still alive is a miracle of my heart's adaptability. After one heart operation, the doctor told me that my heart was twice the size of a normal person's. I think it's a miracle that my body adapted to the abnormal circulation of my heart which was always working very hard. Naturally, my heart got bigger and stronger because it worked so hard. I was really surprised at how fantastically the body can adapt. Modern scientific knowledge says that I cannot be alive, but I still am because of my large heart. If my heart had not enlarged itself naturally, I would have died at sixteen. But I couldn't figure out how to cure my heart by macrobiotics. My heart had an extra vein which had to be closed. After I became a mother, I wanted to stay alive, so I tried an operation. After I had my heart operation, George said that I had been foolish. What George said was true, because the vein opened up a year later when I was pregnant with Jiro. Now my condition is the same as a baby in the womb. Even though my heart operation was a success, it made all my organs weak. It took a long time for them to recover. Your physical condition can be changed only by activity, religion or food. If you try to change it with an operation, you lose more than you gain. An operation also involves taking lots of drugs which affect your entire body, especially your nervous system.

Toilet training

It is best to toilet train your child as soon as possible. This is easier to do in the summertime. Set up a schedule of two or four hour intervals. Put the child on the toilet seat and repeat a rhythmical sound, i.e. si, si, si. The sound makes the child relax and urinate quickly. At first, follow the schedule strictly; later the baby will indicate to you by a movement or sound that he has to go to the toilet. I started training my daughter Marie when she was four months old. George Ohsawa said the sooner, the better. Babies don't urinate in their sleep; only when they wake up. As soon as they wake up, bring them to the toilet. In summer, a baby can wear cotton underpants. When he urinates, the pants become wet and cold. This will be an unpleasant feeling for him, so he will learn quickly. When changing the baby's diaper, if the skin is red in color, wash with warm water. Urine contains much salt and acid. This can irritate the baby's skin. If the red color persists this means the baby is uncomfortable, and he usually cries a lot.

Bathing

Normal babies have a red coloring. If they are given a bath every day this takes salt from their skin and allows them to sleep better. Set up a schedule and bathe the baby at the same time every day, except if he is sick. When the baby is three or four months old, begin bathing him before his last feeding. After dinner, the mother has eaten; she relaxes and gives her baby good milk, so he then sleeps a long time. If your baby wakes up two or three times during the night, either the baby is not getting enough milk or the quality is poor. If you are very busy during the day, then you are tired at night. Tired milk is not good for the baby. Rest before or after dinner so you are not so tired. When you are tired, your appetite is also not so good. After six months, it is not necessary to feed the baby at night. The baby will cry, because he is accustomed to eating at a certain time. He will cry perhaps for three successive nights, but after that he will sleep through the night.

Measles

When Marie was two years old and Jiro was one year old, they both caught the measles. My mother was visiting us in New York at that time. She was surprised at Jiro's good appetite. He ate brown rice and mother's milk. My mother said that macrobiotic children were very healthy. In old Japan mothers were very careful when their babies had measles. This was a dangerous disease. It could lead to pneumonia, high fever, sometimes blindness. Babies even died from measles. For macrobiotic children measles is not such a dangerous disease. Do not expose your child to cold drafts; keep him inside. Let the rash cover his body; otherwise it will go internally and cover the organs. Do not give them extreme yin foods such as fruit at this time. George Ohsawa said the cause of measles is that the baby is growing and doesn't need the yang which it received from the mother during pregnancy. Measles is a discharge of excess yang. A yin baby will not have measles until it is yang enough to discharge this excess yang. Usually a baby has measles between the ages of two to four. Do you know if your baby has a yin or yang condition?

Social training

The second time George Ohsawa came to the United States, he stayed in my home. At that time, Marie and Jiro were both walking, so he took them to Central Park for a walk. Later he said to me, "Cornellia, my grandchildren not so good. People in the park talk to them, they say 'Hello' or 'How cute' but your children don't respond. Everybody loves children," he said. "You must educate your children to be open to everyone, not to be exclusive." It is better to train your children to be yang, friendly and active, than to be yin and timid. When we moved to Chico, I made friends with more American macrobiotics and learned from them. America is the country of individualism; we think of ourselves first, then others. One of my friends had a baby at home. I went to cook for her in her home with my children. My friend's husband once gave his children bread, but not my children, even though we were staying in the same house. Japanese people do not make this discrimination. They try to treat all children alike and share things equally among them. Americans make the distinction "mine" and "yours." When everyone is treated in like manner, this is oneness. This is very important to practice in our life. If you really understand the Unique Principle then your life is always oneness—you and I are the same, not separate. All aspects of your daily life will flow smoothly when you practice oneness and nonexclusivity; this will not be taught in school or by books. Parents must show their understanding of oneness by their life to their children. If your life shows your understanding of oneness, it is integrating. Then you really recognize the miracle of living. When you realize the oneness in your life, then your life is full of gratitude and freedom.

In Japan, they say what you are at three years of age, you will be even when you are 100 years old, because of the education your parents gave you. Until a child is three, good and bad must be clearly defined. Emphasize flexibility. Discipline is strong and consistent. Good manners, care of material things are taught to the child by the mother. One has to be a good mother, because the child learns from your example. To develop strength, a big dream, and health in your children, keep them seven percent hungry and three percent cold. It is very difficult to be seven percent hungry if you are not poor. However, other children eat sugar and tropical fruits, but a macrobiotic mother does not give these to her children; this is comparable to seven percent hungry. Love is not giving only;

if your children want sweet food and you do not give it to them, this is a form of love. A mother must show her children a strong will. I say to my children, "Look at my teeth and body; these cannot make a happy life. I don't want you to have such a life, so I don't give you bad food." When your children go to school, special events like parties and holidays arise and they are served sugar cookies and soft drinks. When these events come up, don't make them lie to you. It is most important for them to learn honesty. Tell them to go and enjoy this food. Whatever you eat, it is most important to enjoy it. After eating this food, your children's condition changes, but they must learn this for themselves. While a child is very young, before he goes to school, it is important for him to have an orderly life and good food to make him strong. Even if he eats sugar when he is older, it can cause no great damage. All this depends on your child's condition. If he is active and yang, it is all right but if he is weak and yin, do not give him sugar.

Two years ago, I permitted my children to go out on Halloween. They collected lots of candy. For that night, I allowed them to eat candy, but the next day I gave all that was left to the neighbor's children. They miss not eating candy; sometimes they even hide candy in their room. I advise them to continue eating macrobiotic food until they are sixteen years old. After that they can decide for themselves what kind of food they prefer. But if they continue to live in my home after sixteen, I won't serve meat or sugar for them. They were born very healthy, so I don't know if they will continue macrobiotics or choose another way. To me, it seems they must judge for themselves. A child's life is not yours; they must choose for themselves and make their own way. I give them complete freedom after sixteen.

In day-to-day life, we should impress our children with honesty and earnestness. Each day we should be making a better day, so our children will have happy memories of the time spent with their parents and friends.

Baby and salt

Babies born on a macrobiotic diet are usually healthy and immune to many sicknesses. During pregnancy if the diet is too yin or too yang, or if drugs are taken, the unborn child receives the mother's imbalances and toxins. If this occurs, when the baby is born it will be weak and crave salt. It is all right to give the baby miso, tamari, gomashio, etc., in small quantities. However, do not give raw salt.

"To determine whether your baby needs salt," George Ohsawa said, "give him a large piece of daikon pickle (about two or three inches long). If he needs salt, he will suck on it all day long, but if he has enough salt, he will leave it alone." This is a very good snack for babies. Since most macrobiotic Americans grew up on a diet of meat, they cannot take much salt. Their babies, however, are macrobiotic, so their condition is different from their own. Often parents are afraid to give their baby salt. Some mothers think that it is good to feed their baby lots of fruit. For the mother, her body is adapted to this, but the baby's body is made from a grain and vegetable diet. So the baby will become anemic if he is fed lots of fruits and vegetables without salt (including miso or soy sauce). These foods can also produce parasites in the baby's body. Too much salt is also bad for the baby. If you mistakenly feed your baby too much salt, give him water. This takes salt from the body. Salt is important in our blood. The Japanese word for blood is "chishio;" "shio" means salt. Please study more the relationship between salt and your baby. If he eats enough salt, then a baby will have a deep sleep and cry very little. The Japanese say that sleep helps the baby to grow better. When a baby sleeps deeply, he grows at an even pace. A mother should drink a third of a cup of bancha tea after each meal and urinate three or four times a day. This shows her condition is good. If she is more thirsty, then her cooking is too salty or else she eats too many side dishes. Overeating also makes a mother more thirsty. Too much liquid makes the mother urinate frequently. If you work hard, then the salt you take in goes to your body cells and changes them. If your cells are strong and have the proper amount of salt, you will never get sick. But if your body is weak, mild exercise will help you to build your health quickly.

CHAPTER II

First Solid Foods for Baby

In Japan, when a baby is 100 days old, a celebration is held and the baby is fed solid foods for the first time. For girls this is 110 days. In my home, my father held my younger brother and gave him miso soup from the top of his chopsticks (just a small amount); he put this inside his mouth. Also, he fed him two or three grains of cooked rice. Then the ceremony is over. It is good start the baby on solid foods around this age. If you prefer, you can wait until the baby has two lower and two upper teeth; then they are really ready. Mix raw rice and water (1 to 10). Cook this on a low flame for five hours. This is rice kayu; it is very soft. Mash the rice grains inside the baby's feeding bowl with a spoon and feed this to the baby. Add a little gomashio. Miso soup can also be given, about 1 teaspoon per day at first. Increase this amount gradually. Watch the quantity of salt; do not give the baby too much because he won't take it—he will push the food away instead. Observe the baby's stool for color and consistency. It should be neither too hard nor too soft. It should be firm and smell good. If his stool is green and soft, this indicates too many vegetables or not enough salt. If you feed your baby brown rice every day, it is not necessary to feed him lots of vegetables. Rice contains sufficient minerals for the baby.

When I began to feed Marie solid foods, I fed her soft rice

cream with vegetables. But so much saliva was secreted from her glands, she was always drooling. Later when we went to Europe for six months (we traveled by car for two months), our diet consisted mainly of grains. Then her saliva became normal. I realized that I had been feeding her too many vegetables. Better to feed your baby grains and vegetables separately—not to mix them. If the baby doesn't want vegetables, he will push the spoon out of his mouth. Ojiya, whole wheat or buckwheat noodles and macaroni, all cooked until they are very soft, are easy for the baby to digest. Mochi is a very good food for the baby. Be sure to cut them very small and wet them, so they don't catch on the baby's throat. Cook them with miso soup or clear soup. This is the best solid food for babies, because it stimulates their digestion and promotes vitality and energy. Solid foods do not need to be special foods; just use less salt than for adults.

At one year, a baby should be eating the same variety of food that an adult does. Whole grain is better for the baby than products such as rice cream. If you feed your baby rice cream only, the minerals in the baby's body are affected, since rice cream is a flour product. Gradually they lose their vitality. Chewed brown rice is the best food for your baby. Some babies don't like cooked carrots and onions; these vegetables are too yang for them. The baby reacts this way instinctively. If your baby eats lots of carrots, his condition is yin. If your baby won't eat cooked vegetables, don't use oil. Instead try this method. Put a piece of kombu on the bottom of a pan; on top of it place cut vegetables; half cover these with water and cook until soft; add soy sauce for taste. Feed this to the baby. Some children crave salt. When this happens, give it to them. The mothers of these babies often took lots of drugs, so the baby's body has taken in all these toxins from the mother. These babies have a very yin condition, so they crave salt by instinct. A friend of mine forced her children to eat gomashio even though they didn't want it. I told her to stop this and be guided by her children's intuition. In this case, feeding them too much salt made the children stutter.

In Japan, women feed their babies breast milk but forget about water. A few months after birth, it is good to give your baby a little water also. This can be done with a teaspoon. If the baby doesn't want it, don't force him. Often a baby cries even though the mother has sufficient milk. If this happens, give the baby some water. At the New York summer camp, Jiro was drooling a lot. We gave him less water. He went by the lake and began to drink stagnant water from an old boat. He was very small and could only wet his fingers and suck this water from his fingers. I brought him to the kitchen and gave him a glass of well water. He smiled and fell into a deep sleep. From this time, I never denied water to my children, unless they began to sneeze or had a runny nose. In Chico, a friend of mine had two babies; both were very inactive. That year the Foundation had a summer camp in Big Sur. George Ohsawa was there. He looked at these children and said that the trouble was too much salt and not enough water. He advised a salt-free diet for both children. After a few days, they lost all excess from their bodies by sneezing, drooling and a runny nose. Then they became more active, began to walk. If your child doesn't smile or doesn't cry, this indicates too much salt. It is easy to remedy this, because excess salt can be eliminated quickly. At that time, I was in Japan. When I returned home I was surprised to see my friend's children. Now they had worms, because they had followed a salt-free diet for a long time. I recommended an increase in salt intake and to feed them buckwheat. Soon the worms were gone from their bodies. If your children eat too much fruit, sugar or honey, they make their condition yin. To change this to a yang condition takes time, because these foods have taken minerals and calcium from the body. A baby will feel bad, he will always cry and never smile.

If a baby eats grain, gradually he will have only one bowel movement per day. A golden brown color is best. If you feed him many green vegetables, sometimes this makes the stool green in color. This is all right as long as it smells good and is neither too soft nor too hard. Urine should be yellow; if it has no color, feed your baby more salt. After five months of age a baby can be given salt; only a little bit. Rice crackers, bread crust or mochi arari are good snacks. Oblong-shaped rice balls are also good. Solid foods are nothing special to prepare, so a mother can enjoy this time. Macrobiotic children have strong stomachs and intestines, so everything is digested well. If your child doesn't want some particular food, don't give it to him. When you follow the macrobiotic diet strictly, you will naturally know the right amount of salt for your child. I have remembered many of the teachings of George Ohsawa in my article; if they have helped you in any way, I'm very happy.

CHAPTER III

Prenatal and Postnatal Care

Around the ninth month of pregnancy, the baby's head is down because the brain is growing and the weight of it pulls downward. If a baby's head is up instead of down, the brain is not completely grown. "This is abnormal," George Ohsawa said. At this time, the mother will urinate frequently because of the pressure on the bladder caused by the baby's head. When you urinate, put your hands under the baby's head and lift up; urination will be easier. Sometimes pregnant women have trouble with swollen legs. At this time, reduce your salt intake or your intake of yin foods. When the labor pains are five minutes apart, braid your hair in two braids (if it is long). After the baby's birth, don't comb your hair for one week. When you comb your hair, your energy goes to your head, and sometimes you become flushed. This is not good. If you have a long labor, it is all right to eat a snack if you feel hungry. Shoban is good, but if it is too salty it will make the birth canal contract. During pregnancy, if you have eaten well macrobiotically (a little bit of fruit or the white part of fish or carp is all right if you crave it) and maintained an orderly life, the birth will be quick and breast milk will come naturally.

After the baby's birth, keep your head low—maybe sleep without a pillow. Your movements should be slow; don't get up or sit down quickly. The blood circulation is difficult after birth and you may become dizzy. If you rest properly, your recovery will be quicker. Completely rest in bed for at least three days. Only get up to go the bathroom. In old Japan, a new mother stayed in bed and didn't go outside for at least three weeks. If you take proper care of yourself now after the birth of the baby, then later you will have an easier time during your change of life. If your change of life period is very difficult, it is because you didn't take proper care of yourself after giving birth. For the next day after giving birth, eat kayu with salt plums, vegetable miso soup and unyeasted bread. Simple food is best for recovery and to strengthen your womb. Thereafter, regular food can be eaten. Three weeks before the birth of the baby, cease sexual activity. Otherwise the water breaks too soon and delivery is very difficult on the mother. If your husband is yang and cannot wait, have him try this exercise. He should breathe deeply from his abdomen (hara) ten times and his sexual desire will change to father's love. After birth, refrain from sexual activity for three weeks.

Congratulations on the birth of your baby

After birth, cover the baby's body with a receiving blanket. Clean the baby's eyes with cotton balls dipped in warm water. Cover your index finger with gauze, wet it with warm water and clean out the inside of the baby's mouth. Wash the head with warm water. Draw a bath for the baby. Measure the temperature with your elbow. If it is not too hot, then it is a good temperature. Place the baby's head on your left arm and with your left hand hold the baby's left hand. Place your right thumb on the baby's anus. This prevents him from having a bowel movement in the bath. Slowly immerse the baby into the bath. When the baby relaxes, remove your thumb from his anus and remove the receiving blanket. Wash his neck, underarms, sexual organs, and then legs. After the front is washed, roll the baby over. Hold the baby's right hand in your left. Wash his back and anus. Then the bath is finished. Wet a small piece of gauze with warm water and hold it in the baby's mouth for awhile. If he is a normal yang baby, he will not need to eat for one day. The mother can rest completely. When her breasts fill with milk, then feed the baby. At first, the milk will have no color. It will be a little oily. This acts as a laxative to clean out the baby. It is very important to feed this milk to the baby first. The baby will have a black stool—this is normal. If the baby doesn't have this black stool, it will have difficulties as an adult.

Visiting

Friends shouldn't visit a new mother until a week after the baby's birth. To send gifts is all right. If you visit during the first week, just see the baby and mother for a short time, be quiet, and then leave. Once I visited a friend the week after she gave birth. I found her very tired and unable to sleep. She was pale, but her head was hot. She had too many visitors. The day before, her friend came with three children. They were very active children and they stayed a long time, exhausting the new mother. Even in a hospital you can only visit for a set time twice a day. I advised her husband to use apple juice for a compress. Until it was ready I placed my hand on her forehead and spoke softly to her. I brought her some carp soup because her husband told me that the baby always cried. From birth, the baby had not been bathed, because the parents didn't know how to bathe the baby. I gave the baby a bath. I discovered a three inch piece of plastic on the baby's navel which had been used to stop the blood during birth. It was irritating the baby, so he cried. After giving the baby a bath, I fed carp soup to the mother. Both mother and baby fell asleep for five hours. A baby who is yang by birth needs a bath to remove excess salt. Then he falls into a deep sleep.

People who give birth at home need to know how to bathe the baby. For the first week an experienced friend or the husband should bathe the baby once a day, preferably in the afternoon. After one week the mother can do this. At first it is difficult to handle the baby, but with practice you soon learn. Bath time is a good opportunity to observe the baby's body.

New babies perspire often so the areas of the neck, under-arms and sexual organs become dirty quickly and need to be cleaned daily. If the diaper area is red, apply vegetable oil and baby powder. Before a bath, take off all the baby's clothes except his undershirt and diaper. Cover his body and take the baby to the bathroom. Put a small mat on the floor. Lie the baby down. Draw a basin of warm water. Clean his eyes, face, then head. When washing the head, hold the baby. Soap is not necessary. Put elbow temperature water in the baby's bathtub, take off his diaper and undershirt, cover his body with a receiving blanket so that the baby doesn't slip into the water. Follow the same procedure as you did at birth. A yang baby even in cold weather doesn't need a lot of clothes. Cotton clothes are best next to the skin; woolen clothes are not good for babies. Clothes should not bind, since babies move their arms and legs a lot.

Breast feeding

Every three hours breast feed your baby, but it is not necessary to wake him if he is sleeping. Soon you will discover which cry is from hunger. When the baby is satisfied it will stop sucking. If the baby dozes while eating and is not eager to eat, it is better to leave the baby in the crib and not to feed him. If the baby isn't satisfied, at the next feeding he will eat eagerly. A feeding should last no more than twenty minutes. If the baby plays while eating, then it is also better to leave him in the crib. In the beginning, it is important to train the baby so he doesn't take too much of the mother's time. The mother should train the baby well so it won't be spoiled. After you have been macrobiotic about three years, your skin becomes tougher. Otherwise the skin around the nipples will crack. To make the skin stronger pinch the nipples lightly or rub them with a dry washcloth. George Ohsawa said, "Macrobiotic cooks should not remove skins from vegetables; this makes your own skin stronger."

It is not necessary to use soap when bathing—use a rice bran bag. After the birth of a baby, take care not to shock the new mother. A shock can completely stop the mother's milk. My aunt's third child was born with a blue mark on its forehead. A friend told her this was a permanent mark. She was so shocked, she had no more milk. Even though she had another baby, she had no milk. She had to feed her baby rice milk. If you have sufficient breast milk, but argue with your husband, this changes the quality of your milk; it becomes more acid. You must establish peaceful surroundings to insure the quality of your milk. Squeeze your breast and test the drop of milk that comes out on your fingernail. If it runs off, the milk is too watery; you are too yin. It should retain its form. This indicates good quality milk. If your milk will not come out of your breasts (usually because the hole is closed off), this means you are too yang. Stop eating all animal protein. Apply a ginger compress, followed by an albi plaster. George Ohsawa said that even a sick mother's milk is better than cow's milk. You must improve the quality of your milk by good food, so your baby will be healthy.

A deep sleep is essential for smooth growing of the baby. A baby is born small and it grows bigger. This is normal. A red, yang baby drinks mother's milk which is sweet and liquid (yin), so it grows quickly. If your baby's color is pink or white, use more yang food in your diet and the baby will become normal naturally. A proper amount of sea salt and activity will produce a healthy baby. If you don't do any hard work, you cannot take salt. A baby's cry should be loud. This means the lungs are well developed and strong. However, this doesn't mean that a baby should always be crying. A baby cries from hunger, a wet diaper, or pain.

Mother's warmth

Before I had my own children, I had little experience with babies. Both my children were born in the United States, so my way is American. Both children slept in cribs. Marie always sucked her pillow. Jiro always sucked his baby blanket. This is uncommon in Japan. A baby after birth is always at his mother's side. He feels his mother's warmth. When a baby starts to crawl, a mother puts him on her back so he is always in contact with warm skin. These babies never suck pillows or blankets. When you cook, it is better for the baby to stay in the crib. I used to bring Marie into the kitchen and always talked to her while I cooked. At the New York summer camp, George Ohsawa scolded me. "Don't bring babies into the kitchen," he said. This is good advice. Children can injure themselves in the kitchen. Always try to keep your children quiet when you are working. After my heart operation, while I was resting, Marie often made lots of noise, but if I was busy cleaning the house, then she was very quiet. I'm not sure if the Japanese or the American way is better, because my children sucked their blankets and pillows. I tried to raise my children the American way; to be strong and independent. But also I held them very little because this was the way George Ohsawa taught.

Boys and girls have different physical conditions. When Marie was two months old, I stopped breast feeding her. Our landlord took care of her. When I went out, Marie always said "Good-bye"—she didn't cry. After Marie's birth, I caught a cold. I knew my life would be short now, so I gave her a lot of my love. One-third of my weight changed to breast milk. In this way, I gave my love to her. I tried to make her understand the depth of motherly love, even though she would have no mother. Fortunately, I am still alive, but Marie received that mother's love so she wasn't so attached to me. Jiro, I breast fed for thirteen months. A baby boy needs to be held more, but I didn't hold my son. I wanted him to be independent, so I kept a separation between mother and son. Maybe he needed more love. He always cried when I left home. When my children were 4 and 5 years old, they went to Japan for one year with a friend. Jiro cried; he wanted to stay with me. Marie, whose eyes were filled with tears, said to Jiro, "Mommy said we must go to Japan to study Japanese. Next year our mommy will come for us." I was surprised; she was so mature for her age.

She was a good older sister. I'm very grateful to macrobiotics.

Later, we moved to Chico, which is very different from New York City. The house was colder than New York, so when the children got up early in the morning, after they went to the bathroom, they did not return to their own beds, but to mine. Marie was very quiet, she waited until I woke up. But a mother and child are very sensitive to each other, so her presence woke me. I brought her into my bed. Jiro was much different. He stamped his feet very loudly and complained that he was cold. When he saw Marie in my bed, he became jealous and felt that Marie was my favorite. With Marie on my right and Jiro on my left, they were very happy to spend a short time with me in this way in the morning. Both children had very cold feet so they intertwined their feet in my legs; they were very happy because they became warm. Herman felt I was spoiling them and he said he couldn't sleep, so I shouldn't do this. I felt they needed their mother's warmth and since they were in bed for such a short time, it was all right. American children do not go to their parents' bed. I still remember my mother's warmth. I was a sick child, so I always slept with my mother. Jiro slept with me until he was six; Marie was five. I think boys need mother's love more than girls—maybe because their physical condition is yin. I cannot say whether the American or the Japanese style is better. But parent-child relationships among the Japanese are more warm and affectionate. A child always feels the mother's warmth. His body remembers the warmth of his mother's body. I think it is a good practice for children to stay in bed with their mother because they all relax. American babies are fed cow's milk and are kept separate from their mother, so they don't feel her warmth. This creates the individualism here in America. For the benefit of the child's character, a mother should give her child a lot of attention until he is three years old. If this is sufficient, later the children won't be dependent on the mother's physical presence. My mother didn't breast feed me. Because of that, her father-in-law told her that her relationship with me was not warm enough. So she carried me on her back so I could feel her warmth. My mother was very yang and temperamental. She wouldn't eat leftover food from her baby's feeding. She felt this was dirty. Still, she loved children very much and she listened to her father-in-law, so her children love her deeply.

On the American frontier, the relationship between parents and children must have been closer. Mothers breast fed their babies—the baby felt the mother's warmth. Now we have many material conveniences. Children have their own rooms; central heating controls heat and cold, so it is not necessary for the child to know the mother's warmth. Also, the convenience foods are much different than mother's own cooked food. Mother's cooking is full of love and attention. Macrobiotic children are very lucky. Our children can go out and distribute their happiness to the world. I hope all macrobiotic children do this. Children need to have social awareness which only the mother can teach. If a mother is selfish and concerned only with her family, the children will be the same. A mother must always have a big dream; make everyone around her happy, not just her family. Macrobiotic children are very special; they have been given a great gift. Their mothers must educate them not to be selfish but to be concerned with everyone in the world: to make everyone healthy, happy and free. I covered many topics in my article; if they can help you at all, I am very happy.

CHAPTER IV

Diseases and Treatments

How to distinguish disease

Observe when fever begins: morning, afternoon or evening. This is one way to identify yin or yang sickness. A hot afternoon sun (yang) draws out excess yin from the body. This causes fever. Both night and early morning are yin, so excess yang comes out. TB patients usually experience fever in the afternoon; TB is a very yin sickness. Fever in the morning is caused by excess yang (animal food).

Usually, constipation comes with sickness. When my children were small I would check their stools every day. This way I could tell easily if their diet was too yin or too yang. If children are constipated, please give them an enema. When bowels are clean, fever will not come and the body will be strong.

In hot summer, babies become constipated easily. To help baby have a bowel movement, cut a cabbage core into a triangular shape and insert between buttocks two or three times.

Using macrobiotic remedies there is no danger of hurting the child. If you make a mistake as to yin or yang cause of sickness, no harm is done—except in a life or death situation. If a yang remedy doesn't work, then try a yin remedy. Mother just needs to be observant.

If you use drugs to cure sickness, serious problems can arise.

Wax on baby's head

Two months after the baby is born, a wax-like skin disease may develop on the baby's head. This wax is a discharge of animal protein accumulated in the womb and from breast feeding. This discharge will help the baby grow strong. Do not put external medicines on the head. They will stop the discharge and damage the kidneys.

After I had my son Jiro I was very weak. I ate some salty pickled salmon which made my milk very yang. Jiro developed head wax one month later.

If your baby is breast feeding and has this wax it is a good idea to stop taking all animal food. Head wax takes six months to one year to finish, depending on the quantity of animal food the mother has taken.

To remove head wax, bathe the head with warm water and rice bran bag to soften the wax. Then, put sesame or olive oil on the head and gently wipe off the wax with a cloth. You may also use this to wash the baby instead of soap. Rice bran protects the body from all skin diseases. To make a rice bran bag:

> Fill a cotton cloth with rice bran and tie it into a bag. Soak in hot water for a few minutes. The bag is ready to use when a whitish liquid can be squeezed through the cloth.

Bed wetting

Sometimes macrobiotic children wet the bed. The cause can be either an expanded or a contracted bladder. If the child wets the bed soon after going to sleep, it is a yin cause. The child becomes warm in bed and the bladder relaxes. When the child wets the bed in the early morning, the cause is too yang. The parasympathetic nervous system is active at this time and it squeezes an already contracted bladder.

To yangize an expanded bladder (yin cause):

Mix 70% kohren (dried lotus root) with
30% black gomashio (sesame salt made
with black sesame seeds), 9:1.

Put this in a capsule and give it to the child before bed. Also,
give 1 teaspoon black gomashio at each meal. To yinnize a
contracted (yang) bladder, give mochi and Chinese cabbage.
Any white vegetable is good. Also, give less salt.

Diaper rash

My children never had diaper rash because I never gave
them fresh fruit. I think too much fruit produces acid in the
urination. This is the cause of diaper rash. If you are breast
feeding your baby and it develops a rash, cut down your intake of fruit.

To relieve pain from a diaper rash: each time you change
diapers, wash the infected area with warm water, then dry
and cover the rash with sesame oil and corn starch.

Tonsilitis

Symptoms of tonsilitis are sore throat, excessive saliva in
the mouth and high fever. The most important treatment is to
break any high fever that develops as it can damage the kidneys. Then you can use a salt plaster to cure the tonsilitis.

To make a salt plaster:

Use 1 or 2 cups of sea salt and add
enough water to dampen it—between 3
and 7 tablespoons.

Put the salt on a 10 x 24″ thin cotton cloth. Roll this and wrap
it around the child's neck. Cover the plaster with a dry hand
towel, securing it with a safety pin. Leave this on overnight.
Remove it in the morning and clean the neck with warm
water. This treatment is good for adults also.

Four years ago a student of mine, thirty years old, complained of having had periodic pain in her throat for three years. I gave her salt plaster and overnight she was cured. Western doctors take out the tonsils but this is not necessary and will not decrease throat infections. George Ohsawa said, "Never take out the tonsils." I think tonsils control and produce hormones and are very necessary to good health.

Stuffy nose

Babies cannot blow a stuffy nose, so mother must help. With her mouth she can gently suck mucus from each nostril. As a remedy, cut one inch from a white scallion stem and put in a nostril for twenty minutes. Remove and put a fresh piece in the other nostril.

For an older child or an adult you can use a bancha tea/salt remedy:

Mix together ½ teaspoon sea salt, ⅓ cup
hot bancha tea and ⅔ cup of water.

Close a nostril and inhale some of the liquid into the other nostril. Blow out into a basin of water. Do the same with the other nostril. If the excreted mucus sinks, the congestion is caused by ozena, a disease of the mucus membranes. Use the bancha/salt mixture every day until the sinus cavity is clear. Avoid sugar, fruits and animal products if you have congestion.

Infection on inside of mouth

Breast-fed babies do not usually have this trouble. If it occurs, habu-cha will cure it. Habu-cha is an herb tea available in Japanese stores. To prepare it:

Add 1 heaping tablespoon habu-cha to 1
cup of water. Boil in a porcelain pot for
20 minutes. Strain and immerse 3 cotton

balls in the liquid. Wipe the inside of the baby's mouth three times, once with each ball.

Skin disease

Rub sliced daikon on affected area and cover with sesame oil. Wash the baby with a rice-bran bag instead of soap. All skin diseases are caused by weak kidneys. Sugar, fruit and animal products will aggravate the condition.

Bee Stings

Chew bancha leaves (any green tea leaves will work) and put over the sting area. This will relieve the pain quickly. Children and adults who are stung by bees frequently have high blood sugar content (hyperglycemic, diabetic). These people produce a sweet smell like fruit or sugar which attracts bees and other insects.

Mosquito bites

Mix dentie with your saliva and rub on the bite. This will help the itching and prevent infection. If your child eats sweet foods, many mosquitos will be attracted.

Nose bleed

With the side of your palm hit the back of the neck three times. Sit with head slightly forward and block bleeding nostril. Hold for a few minutes and breathe through the mouth.

Occasional nose bleeds are common with children and not a serious problem; however, if bleeding is very heavy and doesn't stop in a few minutes, contact a doctor. Also, if nose bleeds are frequent—consult a doctor.

Curing colds

There are many causes and symptoms of colds. A child who has coughing and mucus discharge is suffering from chest cold. The cause is yin. A good treatment is lotus root soup. Lotus root is white and watery. It grows in swamps and spreads its roots horizontally under the soil. So it has both yin and yang qualities. To make lotus root soup:

Mix 1 tablespoon grated lotus root, ¼ teaspoon grated ginger and a touch of sea salt in ½ cup boiling water.

The health of a baby will suffer if it is exposed to cold on its stomach. This can occur from kicking its blanket off at night or being near a cold draft. The baby will develop a cold with light coughing and low fever. This is like a summer cold. Eating fruits will also cause this condition as they will make the stomach cold and inhibit digestion. Fruits kill enzymes in the intestines so body will not make good quality blood. Daikon, shiitake and lotus root will not help this type of yin cold. I recommend scallion miso soup, as it kills harmful stomach bacteria and warms the stomach and intestines. To prepare:

Bake 1 tablespoon miso on top of the stove, using either a dry, uncovered skillet or a metal toaster (available in Japanese stores), until brown. Mix ⅓ of the miso with 1 heaping tablespoon of the white root part of scallion. Add 1 cup boiling water.

For a cold with sore throat, coughing, fever, headache and mucus discharge I recommend three-vegetable soup. To make three-vegetable soup:

Use 4 or 5 shiitake mushrooms, 2 pieces fresh lotus root sliced ⅓″ thick, and 2

pieces daikon, same size. Cook in 2 cups
of water for 1 hour over a low flame.
Strain and add a little tamari.

Give this in ½ cup servings at intervals until the fever is
down and misery is relieved.

Fever

To lower a high fever quickly I recommend sour apple
juice. If the fever is over 102°, boil the juice slightly. Also
good for lowering fever are Chinese cabbage, daikon and
scallion cooked into soup.

Fever over 102° is usually caused by the toxins from animal protein—fish, red meat, eggs, cheese, etc. Number One
daikon soup is good for neutralizing these toxins. It will
induce sweating and break the fever. To prepare:

Mix 1 tablespoon grated daikon, ⅓ teaspoon grated ginger, ½ teaspoon tamari
and 1 cup hot bancha tea.

Serve to child. After giving the soup, keep the child warm in
blankets for 20 minutes. The soup will induce sweating and
break the fever. Give daikon soup often until the fever stays
down.

Fever accompanied by depression, hysteria and uncon-
trollable behavior is often caused by blood stagnation in the
head. This too is caused by animal protein. Shiitake mush-
room soup is good for breaking up stagnated blood. To
prepare:

Place 3 dried shiitake mushrooms in 2
cups water, bring to boil and simmer
30 minutes. Strain and add 1 teaspoon
tamari.

This will quiet the child and lower the fever.

Tofu plaster can also be used for fever of the head.

Squeeze excess liquid from tofu, mix with flour, wrap in cheese cloth and apply to head. For head injury from car accident, fall, etc., shave hair around the wound, hollow out a cabbage, fill with tofu and put over injury. This will keep the head cool and prevent blood from stagnating. It is the fever and blood stagnation after the injury that causes brain damage in many cases.

Sore throat

When the child has a sore throat, give kuzu soup with kombu charcoal mixed in. It is the kombu charcoal that soothes the throat. The kuzu helps the charcoal stick to the throat rather than go down into the stomach where it can't help the throat. Kombu charcoal helps cure the infection which causes the pain. It is also good for intestines and weak stomach. For kombu charcoal, see "Charcoal Medicines."

Any kind of disease weakens the stomach and intestines. They must be treated and made strong for the body to cure itself.

Cough

One year ago a woman phoned about her one-year-old boy. She said he is a very active boy but has a persistent cough. She had given him much goat milk, which is very yang. I advised her to give him yinnie syrup juice. (To obtain yinnie syrup, order from Chico-San, Inc., P.O. Box 1004, Chico, CA 95927.) To prepare:

> Slice 5 or 6 pieces daikon ¼" thick, place in a glass jar and cover with 1 cup yinnie syrup. Let sit 1 hour. A clear juice will come to the top of the jar. This is yinnie juice.

One day later the mother called again. Yinnie juice didn't stop the cough but did improve his appetite. I advised her to try Number 2 daikon soup; later I received a nice card saying the daikon soup cured the cough. To prepare:

Make ½ cup daikon juice by grating daikon and squeezing through cheesecloth. Mix with ½ cup water and slightly boil (simmer).

These are good proportions for a baby.

Number 2 daikon soup is good for organs of the urinary system and to lower fever. It also dissolves old salt in the body.

Stomach trouble

A baby's stomach sits vertically in the abdomen; when he overeats, the excess is vomited easily. As the child grows, the stomach shifts to a horizontal position, making it easier to overeat.

A good medicine for stomach trouble is umeboshi plum or ume extract (concentrated plum with no salt). Ume is also good for fever and diarrhea. Give an azuki bean size portion two or three times a day. Dissolve the ume in a small quantity of warm bancha tea or water. Ume extract has a very strong effect on body germs. About five years ago in Seattle a four-year-old boy died suddenly and I then discovered it was from dysentery and that the rest of the family also had it. So I told them and all their friends' children to take plum concentrate with umeboshi because you can cure dysentery and diarrhea that way. (George Ohsawa said that dysentery is caused by fruit, and the American diet often includes a lot of fresh fruits, pies, etc.) The whole family in Seattle was cured in about 10 days with rice kayu, plum extract and umeboshi. When a baby has these ailments and his feet are cold, keep them warm with a hot bottle. I would recommend that if you have a child, keep a bottle of the extract around.

(To order umeboshi plums and ume extract, write: Soken Trading Co., Box 1705, Sausalito, CA 94965.)

As an external treatment for stomach problems use yaki shio (roasted salt). To prepare:

Roast 1 - 4 cups of sea salt in a dry skillet for 5 minutes on a medium high flame. Put the hot salt in a cotton cloth and tie it shut.

Place this on the baby's stomach over a thin towel or cloth. Be careful the salt pack is not too hot.

A salt pack is also good for treating earaches.

When a baby has stomach trouble and has no appetite, do not force it to eat, but wait for the appetite to return. When the baby's appetite returns, give it rice cakes (such as Chico-San rice cakes). If it has fever and diarrhea and is often thirsty, give bancha tea or cooled boiled water. A friend of mine works as a nurse in a Belgian hospital. She treats many cancer patients and recommends well-chewed rice cakes and very little liquid intake.

The best treatment for intestinal gas is charcoal umeboshi (see "Charcoal Medicines"). It is a very yang medicine and it keeps the body warm. Mix charcoal umeboshi with kuzu soup and the child will become warm quickly. To externally warm the baby, use a hot water bottle. Do not use an electric blanket. It gives off yin vibrations and dries the skin's natural oils.

Diarrhea

There are two causes of diarrhea, yin and yang. Yang diarrhea is caused by very active intestines. All food is passed through the body very quickly. The stool color is yellow. Yin diarrhea is caused by weak, expanded intestines. Stool color is green, with mucus. To treat yang cause of diarrhea, give grated raw apple, then baked apple. For yin cause, give kuzu soup with charcoal umeboshi.

Constipation

Yang constipation is caused by too much meat, eggs and salt. Give one teaspoon sesame oil, and then give an enema.

Yin constipation is caused by expanded intestines. Use roasted salt pack on intestines and give an enema with warm salted water.

As a general treatment for weak and tired digestive organs, give ume-sho-bancha tea. It also helps poor circulation, weak heart and fatigue. I recommend it after a hot bath to replace body salts. Ume-sho-bancha is good when fasting, as it helps to pass old stools. It is also good for women in labor.

I had an operation on my gums. Afterwards I took ume-sho-bancha tea three times during the night. I had no pain and recovered quickly. My recipe for ume-sho-bancha:

> Use ½ umeboshi plum, ⅓ teaspoon tamari and 2 - 3 drops ginger juice. Mix into ½ cup of hot bancha tea.

For a stomach ache, a ginger compress is effective. To make a ginger compress you need:

> ⅓ cup grated ginger, 10 cups boiled water, 3" x 4" cotton bag, 2 hand towels, 1 pair rubber gloves, portable hot plate. Grate ginger, put in cotton bag and tie shut. Put bag in the hot water. Stir the bag with a chopstick until juice appears in the water. Leave bag in the water.

Fold two towels to size of stomach and place in the hot ginger water. With rubber gloves on, wring the towels and place over the child's stomach. Be careful they do not burn the skin. When one towel cools, change it. In 10 to 15 minutes the stomach will become red as blood is drawn to the stomach to cleanse it.

If you have a portable hot plate, use it to keep the water hot. Do not boil the ginger water, as it will kill the ginger enzymes. Use the same ginger water two or three times a day, each time adding 1 tablespoon of grated ginger to the bag.

CHAPTER V

How To Be a Beautiful and Loved Wife

Natural beauty

Before marriage, I went to school and had a job, so I always wore make-up. I got married when I was thirty years old. I realized I was getting old. One day my husband asked me whether I thought lipstick and make-up made me beautiful. He said, "Look at the squirrels in the park, how cute they are; they have natural beauty." January 15 is Japanese women's New Year. For that occasion I dressed in a kimono (it takes about thirty minutes to put one on). My husband said to me, "If you have time to put on a kimono, then you have time to study more English. I would be happier if you studied English." I was very happy for my husband's remarks. He is like a traditional man. I have a very good husband, but I had two children very close together, also many visitors and much work so I didn't pay attention to my appearance, especially my clothes. But I still use lipstick everyday, because it makes my face seem more alive. I have a very plain face.

My mother came to visit us in New York City. Now I was able to go and help my husband in his store. The first time I went there, he laughed and said to me, "You look like you are wearing your grandmother's clothes." Another Japanese girl, married to an American, also worked there. She was a beautician by profession, so she was always very well made up and stylish. She told me she was very happy that my husband said he would take her when he goes to Japan for business. I was very surprised. I didn't know this. I didn't have much time to talk to my husband; he woke up at 9:00 in the morning, went to the store at noon and came home at 2:00 in the morning.

However, the following Sunday, I discussed many things with him. I asked him about this girl, but he said he forgot he said that to her. He didn't realize how hurt I had been. Shortly after this, we had to leave the country; we went to Europe with the children. We traveled for six months and I was able to study many things. I noticed especially the French country girl and how beautiful she was. They were the same age as I, but they wore pink sweaters which brought out their natural coloring. The Japanese way is different. They wear dark colors. They never think of wearing a bright color, even if it makes them look better. I wasn't so concerned about clothes, because I had brought some Japanese kimonos. While traveling, many people invited us for dinner, but sometimes I had to prepare dinner. In a kimono it was difficult. My regular daily clothing was so plain that I was embarrassed to wear it. In Belgium I ordered three dresses to be made for me. I realized that nice clothes improved my appearance. When I returned to the United States, I took better care with my dress.

To cultivate your own natural beauty is most important. Children want their mother to be young and beautiful. One day Jiro said that old people are ugly. I said to him that I'm getting older. After Marie gets married I will be a grandmother. At this Jiro was very upset and he said to Marie that she must not marry, because he didn't want me to be a grandmother. Children don't want their mothers to get old.

Another woman

In Chico, a friend's husband had a girl friend and wasn't coming home. She was pregnant with her second baby and very unhappy. I consulted my husband. He told me that all men are attracted to young and beautiful girls. Men are always active socially, so they have many opportunities to meet young and beautiful girls. However, if his wife has just one thing that she does better than his girl friend, then he will return—i.e. good cook, good housekeeper or has a tender heart. When a husband comes home, if his wife nags him, he will never come back. My friend always complained to her husband; she had no gratitude. I asked my husband if he had a girl friend too. He said that he didn't but he was very attracted to young and beautiful girls. This shocked me; I never realized he was attracted to other women. I never forgot this. If a woman has two or three children and is very busy, she loses her charm. She becomes very practical, not so romantic. George Ohsawa said that women must be beautiful. A woman must understand a man's mentality. So at all times be neat, be clean and look nice.

Seven enemies

A man always develops higher because he works outside the home—he is always being challenged by others. A woman must keep pace with her husband. She must study and learn. This makes her a more vital person. Otherwise her face is like death. Most important, she must understand her husband's work. Always show an interest in his work, so you can have something in common to talk about. You can be an asset for your husband and help him advance in his work. You can invite his fellow workers to your home for dinner.

The Japanese say that when a man works outside the house, he always has seven enemies. So when he comes home, he should be able to relax and be comfortable. He should be like a king at home. Here he can reveal his true self because of his wife's efforts to create a peaceful home for him.

Create a warm home

A wife who thinks of her husband prepares good meals, especially his favorite dishes. A husband receives that love and has the will to go on with his work. Thus, a wife's position is very important. She holds the key to her family's health and happiness. Even if your work is very hard, always be grateful—you will receive rewards. Do not have a disorderly home; prepare appetizing and appealing food, and take care of your appearance. When you are healthy, you wake up earlier than your husband. If you sleep late, your condition is yin. Brush your hair, put on your make-up, iron your clothes. This gives your family the feeling of being awake. Then serve breakfast. When your husband comes home at night, greet and welcome him, because he has been working very hard. Food is an expression of your love. A peaceful dinner relaxes and revives your husband. One day I wasn't home when my husband arrived home. Even though I arrived later and served a dinner which my friend gave me to bring home, my husband was very unhappy. It's important for a wife to be there when her husband comes home and welcome him with a smile. After my heart operation, my body was not very strong. However, I felt I should prepare meals for my husband and his two friends who lived with us. So I made a supper, after which I was completely exhausted. I woke my husband for supper. Later he said to me that he would prepare supper if he could see my smiling face, instead of a tired one. He said that a tired face is worse than tasteless cooking. It is better to have a smiling face and no meal.

I think a man's physical condition is more yin than a woman's, so they need to feel a mother's love. Before marriage he is very sweet to you, but after, he must support you and your children. Sometimes he has many troubles socially, so a man needs a wife who is very warm and loving like his mother.

Sex life

During the day, a woman must conduct herself like an elegant lady, but in the evening she must be like a call girl. A woman must change her manner and thinking many times during the day. George Ohsawa said that if a couple displays too much affection in front of their children, they become preoccupied with love and will never succeed in the world. Never kiss in front of your children. It is not necessary to demonstrate your love outside of the bedroom. A wife can create a soft atmosphere for her husband in the bedroom by her manner—sometimes sweet, sometimes sulky—and especially by the use of perfume. You make yourself a charming wife through tears and sweat. You can always keep the romantic feeling you and your husband had during courtship. Macrobiotic people don't eat meat and sugar so they can enjoy a long sexual life. So study and enjoy your sexual life.

Ugly face

I stayed in the hospital for three years. When I returned home my face was very black in color as a result of many drugs. At home, I began to use rice bran bags to wash my face. These are made by taking a 3 x 5″ piece of porous cotton material. Sew it on two sides, put in 2 heaping tablespoons of rice bran, and tie the top of the bag with a piece of material. Soak this in hot water for a few minutes, then squeeze. A white liquid will appear. Rub your face with this bag. Do this for a week in the morning and evening and you will notice your skin becomes fresher and more alive. Even if you have blemishes, they will not be noticeable. Use a new rice bran bag each time you wash. When you take a bath, soak two rice bran bags and after you have washed with soap, rub your entire body with these bags. Your skin will become as soft as silk. This also protects your skin from disease. To shampoo your hair, seaweed (funori) is the best. Take ⅓ cup of the dried seaweed, mix it with 3 cups of warm water, and bring it to a boil on top of the stove. The seaweed will dissolve. Let it cool to body temperature, put it on your hair and massage it into your scalp. Rinse. Funori gives your hair a natural sheen.

Walking barefoot

Walking barefoot is also very good, especially if you walk early in the morning on the grass when there is still dew. This helps to revitalize you. Also if you have cold feet, this is yangizing for them. Doing this makes the skin on the feet very hard. It may crack, so use a pumice stone (available in Japanese stores) to clean them. It is important to always keep your toes clean, because all organs are connected here by nerves. In Japan on a farm, even though people worked in the field, there was never any sand or dirt in the house. Before they entered the house, everybody washed his feet in a pond and rubbed off the ground-in dirt with a stone. At the entrance of the house there was always a wet cloth for people to wipe their feet. If the wooden floor got dirty, it was immediately mopped.

Women are the flowers of life

When I came home from the hospital, my friends invited us for Thanksgiving dinner. I usually wore slacks, but for this occasion I wore a dress. My son Jiro was so pleased that I looked so nice. I remembered this. Children want their mother to always be young and beautiful. If women were not beautiful, think how sad everyone in the world would be. Let your womanhood blossom out. Take care to look good, smell good. Give men joy with your presence. Give men your energy, your attention. This is a real woman. In our relative life, we call these women flowers of life. Many people, not only her husband, love her. After the long, cold winter, spring comes and the flowers bloom. Life is also the same. After many difficulties pass, then we must blossom into our own individual flowers and realize our own joy. We must be like a flower blossom for our entire life.

One mind, one body

A woman is the center of the house, like the sun is the center of our galaxy. Many troubles come into your life. Please enjoy these difficulties. God gave us a naked body; we are much different than animals who were born with fur. If you keep in mind that you will also leave this world with a naked body, you will not be so concerned with acquiring material possessions. Understand your husband's job, so you can help him and be able to fulfill his needs. A couple's life is one mind, one body. Develop your relationship with your husband to be one mind, one body. A good marriage is not given, but must be created by your effort. In this world, there are about one hundred million men and women who are searching for their better half. You can choose only one from them. Your choice of an ideal better half out of a hundred million is so precious that you must care for him. However, this is not so easy. All of us grow up with different customs and thinking, for twenty years at least. Often a woman has to shed many tears before she attains the happy marriage which she thought would be so ideal when she chose her husband. A happy marriage must be created by the effort of both parties. Without effort, there is no happy marriage, but with effort, an unhappy marriage can be changed to a happy one. Our life is not a round trip. We only have a one-way ticket. It exists to be enjoyed, not to be rejected. Your life is once and for all, and to be enjoyed. I pray for your happy life, and I end my articles.

CHAPTER VI

Recipes for Baby's Food

1. Rice Milk II

If a mother does not have enough milk when nursing, koh-koh is a good substitute. But for some children this is too yang, so rice milk can be used. This is rice milk II, for an infant; rice milk I is for an older baby (see Chapter I). To prepare:

> Place 1 cup brown rice in 10 cups water. Bring to a boil and let simmer 2 - 3 hours. The outer skin of the rice is broken and it turns into a thick juice. Strain out the skin and the liquid left is rice milk. It can be sweetened with amasake or yinnie syrup and it will taste a little bit like mother's milk.

Be careful of yinnie syrup sold in Japanese food stores. Read the label, as it might be made from sweet potato. I recommend Chico-San yinnie syrup, which is made from milled rice, malted barley, and enzymes of malted grains.

2. Soy Milk

Soy milk is very yin and should only be given to yang, healthy babies. In Japan we ate fresh soy beans only during the summer. Soy beans contain much potassium, which helps to cool the body. Soy milk is too yin for macrobiotic mothers during pregnancy because they do not eat meat to balance the high potassium content of soy beans.

A few years ago a family from Holland came to Vega. They had a two-year-old girl who was very skinny, pale and slightly retarded. She could not even sit up by herself. The mother had been giving the baby soy milk. I advised her not to give soy milk and recommended mugwort mochi. Every day we gave the baby two 2" pieces of mochi baked then cooked in miso soup. Three weeks later the baby was sitting by herself, teeth came, she talked, smiled and her cheeks became pink. Mother was so glad.

They made plans to travel to Mexico. All the Vega students and myself were against this. The water in Mexico is not good and the baby's fragile health would suffer. They went anyway. Later I heard that the baby died.

3. Mugwort Mochi

To prepare mugwort mochi:

Soak 7 cups sweet brown rice in 10 cups water for 24 hours. Soak 5 dried mugwort balls in one cup of water overnight. Strain rice. Place a vegetable steamer inside a 6-quart pressure cooker. Bring 2 cups of water to a boil and add the strained rice. Cover and bring to pressure with high flame; when top is jiggling, reduce to medium flame and cook for 30 minutes. Run cold water on outside of pressure cooker to reduce pressure. Add 2 cups hot water and cook for another 30 minutes under pressure. After pressure is normal, turn off flame. Boil the soaked mugwort in soak water for 10 minutes, then strain and shred by hand. Place cooked rice in a metal bowl and mash with a wooden pestle for 20 minutes. Since the rice has become cold, put it back in a vegetable steamer and steam for 10 minutes over a high flame. Add mugwort to the rice and mash again with wooden pestle. Then, form the mochi into balls.

For babies, add mugwort mochi to miso soup.

Mochi can be frozen and will keep for a long time. To prepare frozen mochi, bake it on top of the stove, using a dry skillet or a Japanese toaster, for about 7 minutes or until soft.

Dried mugwort and mugwort mochi can be ordered from Rising Sun Natural Foods, 440 Judah Street, San Francisco, California 94122.

4. Brown Rice Kayu

½ c. brown rice
5 c. water

Rinse rice gently in a pot of cold water. Keep changing the water. Rinse until the water is clear. Cook on a high flame until it boils. Then turn down the flame and cook for 4 - 5 hours. Turn off the heat. Let it sit for 20 minutes. Remove the cover and mix the rice thoroughly before serving.

5. Ojiya (Brown Rice Porridge with Vegetables)

1 c. cooked rice
⅓ c. daikon cut sengiri
¼ c. carrots cut sengiri
3 - 4 c. water

Saute the vegetables in a little bit of oil—first the daikon, then the carrots. Add water and bring it to a boil. Add rice and cook over a low flame for 2 hours. Add miso, soy sauce or salt for seasoning. Cooking without oil is good for the summertime.

6. Suiton (Dumplings in Soup)

Soup
¼ c. cabbage cut sengiri
⅓ c. onion cut sengiri
little bit of carrot
2 c. water
¼ t. oil

Saute onions in oil. Add cabbage and carrot. Cook 5 minutes. Add water and cook for 30 minutes. Add miso or soy sauce and dumplings.

Dumplings
½ c. whole wheat flour
¼ c. buckwheat flour
⅓ c. cold water

Make a batter of these ingredients and drop by spoonfuls into the soup. When dumplings float to the top of the soup, they are done.

7. Rice Cream

Wash rice and toast in a dry pan until it begins to pop and is golden in color. Blend rice at a high speed in a blender or grind it in a flour mill, until it is a fine powder.

½ c. rice cream powder
2 - 3 c. water
pinch of salt

Roast rice cream powder in a dry pan until there is a nut-like fragrance. Mix thoroughly with boiling water. Bring to a boil, then turn down. Cook for 45 minutes to 1 hour. Mix thoroughly before serving.

8. Rolled Oats (Oatmeal)

> 1 c. rolled oats
> 2 - 3 c. cold water
> pinch of salt

Roast oats in a dry pan, stirring constantly, until there is a nut-like fragrance. Add 2 cups of cold water and bring this to a boil. Add cold water again with the salt. After this boils, turn down and cook for 1 - 2 hours.

9. Whole Wheat Spaghetti with Vegetable Soup

> ½ lb. whole wheat noodles
> 1 small onion cut mawashigiri
> 1 medium sized carrot cut in
>   1″ pieces, sengiri
> 2 leaves of cabbage
> 5 c. water
> ¼ t. salt
> ½ t. oil
> 2 T. soy sauce

Cook noodles in a pressure cooker in the following manner. Place noodles in boiling water (100°). The water should come 1 inch above the noodles. Bring up to pressure. Turn off the flame and let sit 15 minutes. Take pan to the sink and pour cold water over the cover until the pressure comes down all the way. Drain off the water and rinse noodles with cold water. Saute onions, cabbage, and carrots in oil, in that order. Add water and bring to a boil. Cover and lower the heat. Cook for 30 minutes, then add salt. Cook 15 minutes more and add soy sauce. Add cooked noodles to soup and bring to a boil. Then it can be served.

10. Macaroni Gratin

> ½ lb. whole wheat macaroni

Bechamel Sauce
1 heaping T. whole wheat pastry flour
2 c. hot noodle water
½ c. milk
½ t. oil
½ t. salt

Cook macaroni as in 11. Heat oil in a pan. Add flour and roast it, stirring constantly until there is a nut-like fragrance. Set it aside to cool. When the flour is completely cool, add milk, noodle water and salt. Bring to a boil. Place the cooked macaroni in a casserole, pour the bechamel sauce over it and bake for 30 minutes in a 350° oven.

11. Whole Wheat Macaroni Soup

½ lb. whole wheat macaroni
4 c. water
½ t. salt

Bring water to a boil. Add the macaroni and salt. Cook for 20 minutes. Drain and let stand. It is not necessary to rinse them with cold water. Just let them cool normally. Then add this cooked macaroni to soup. (Same as in 9.)

12. Mochi made with Rice Flour

5 c. sweet brown rice
7 c. sweet brown rice flour
5 c. water

Rinse rice gently in a pan of cold water. Keep changing the water and wash until the water is clear. Soak for 24 hours with 5 cups of water in a pressure cooker. Place the pot on the stove, using a flame a little higher than medium. When the pressure comes up (the pressure gauge will jiggle), turn the flame down. Cook for 20 minutes. Turn off the heat and let stand for 45 minutes. Mix flour with hot rice and pound with a wooden pestle (suricogi). Then wet both hands with cold water and knead the rice. Knead, wet hands, knead again. Repeat this process because the rice is very hot. When all grains are thoroughly broken down, the kneading process is finished. Now put some water in a steamer pan and bring it to a boil. Put a wet cloth in the pan. When it begins to steam, place the raw mochi on top of this cloth and cover using the same cloth. Cook at a high heat for 20 minutes. Pierce mochi with a dry chopstick. If nothing sticks to it when it is withdrawn, mochi is done. After steaming the mochi, again wet both hands and make 3 inch oblong-shaped balls and cover with some rice flour. Remember to keep your hands wet. Then place these mochi on a cutting board or flat surface to sit for 5 hours. Mochi can also be frozen to be kept for future use. They can be kept this way for a long time. To cook frozen mochi, heat a dry frying pan on top of the stove. Make it very hot. Place mochi on the bottom of the pan. Cover. Cook on a medium flame for 15-20 minutes. Mochi will become soft and a little puffy. Serve with soy sauce, nori or put them into a soup. You can cook any kind of a soup to serve with mochi. This is a good solid food for your baby after he has been weaned or is at least six months old. It is easy for the baby to digest.

13. Miso Zoni (Mochi in Soup)

> 6 pieces of mochi
> ½ bunch scallions cut ⅓" koguchigiri
> ¼ c. daikon
> 3 taro (albi) potatoes
> little bit of carrot
> 1 - 2 T. miso
> 4 c. water

Saute scallions in 1 teaspoon of oil. Add daikon and taro. Then add ¼ teaspoon salt and water. Cook all vegetables until they are tender. Add miso to taste. Put baked mochi into the soup and bring to a boil, then serve.

14. Amasake

Amasake can be made from sweet brown rice, barley, wheat or millet (most any grain).

A. 2 c. sweet brown rice
    4 c. water
    ¼ c. koji

Rinse rice gently in a pan of cold water. Keep changing the water until it is clear. Soak overnight in 4 cups of water. Start flame under the rice a little higher than medium. When pressure comes up, turn flame down and cook rice for 20 minutes. After this, turn off the heat and let stand 45 minutes; cool until the rice can be handled with your hands. Mix koji with the warm rice and allow to ferment 3 - 4 hours. Put the rice in a glass or porcelain bowl when mixing it with the koji. *Do not use a metal bowl.* Keep the rice mixture in a warm place with a cover. During the fermentation period, mix from top to bottom several times until the koji is melted. Then put the mixture in a pan and bring it to a boil. Turn off the heat as soon as one or two bubbles appear. Allow to cool again and put mixture in a glass jar and keep it in the refrigerator. Amasake can be eaten 5-7 days after this. Amasake can be kept for a long time in a cold place if it is cooked over a low flame until it changes to a brown color. Do not use a cover while cooking. This is like sugar and can be used as a sweetening in cakes, karinto, doughnuts, cookies and pies. To serve amasake as a drink, add boiling water and salt. Bring to a boil and serve.

B. 7 c. sweet brown rice flour
    8 c. boiling water
    1 c. koji

Spread sweet brown rice flour on the bottom of a pressure cooker and add boiling water. Mix together well. Bring this mixture to a boil under pressure with a flame slightly higher than medium. When the pressure comes up, turn down and let cook for 20 minutes. Turn off the heat and allow pressure to come down to normal. Cool. Mix together with koji in a glass or porcelain bowl, keep covered in a warm place for 3 - 4 hours. During the fermentation period, mix from top to bottom several times until all the koji is melted. Change the mixture to a casserole dish, put in the oven (350°) with a cover, and bring to a boil. As soon as one bubble appears, remove and cool. Put in a glass jar and keep in refrigerator. This can be eaten 5 - 7 days later. Cook amasake uncovered over a low flame until it has the thickness of apple butter. Use this as a sweetening, with a little bit of lemon rind, in your baking. Amasake used as a filling in crescent rolls is very delicious, especially with lemon rind.

15. Rice Loaf

    4 c. cooked rice
    5 c. warm water
    8 c. whole wheat flour
    2 c. corn meal
    2 c. millet flour
    3 t. (level) salt

Mix ingredients thoroughly. Knead a little bit and let sit overnight covered with a cloth. Heat up the bread pans in the oven, oil and fill pans ⅔ with dough, then cut down the middle with a knife; this keeps loaves from cracking as they expand during the baking. Set in oven with pilot light only, for 1 hour (in electric oven set thermostat as low as possible—about 100°). Next, raise thermostat to 300° and bake for 2 hours or until they test dry.

Food for Sick Baby

Kuzu soup is good when baby's digestion is poor:

Dilute 1 tablespoon kuzu in a small quantity of water. Bring ½ to 1 cup water to a boil and add diluted kuzu. Let simmer a few minutes until the soup becomes a transparent color. Take off heat and add a little tamari. You may add ¼ teaspoon charcoal umeboshi to make soup more yang.

Special rice cream:

Roast 1 cup of rice until it turns brown. Put in 10 cups of water and add ¼ teaspoon sea salt. Cook 2 to 3 hours. Put cooked rice inside cotton cloth and squeeze with rice paddle. The creamy liquid squeezed from the bag is special rice cream. (You can use the leftover rice to make bread.)

Rice kayu:

Add 1 cup of cooked rice to 3 to 6 cups water. Cook until soft and creamy. This is good for children with fever. Noodles and oatmeal are also good for sick children as they are easier to digest than brown rice.

Noodle soup:

Use 1 package udon noodles, 7 leaves Chinese cabbage and 3 scallions. Add udon to 8 cups boiling water, bring to boil and add 1 cup cold water. Bring to boil again. Remove from heat and strain noodles. Chop Chinese cabbage and scallions and put in 8 cups water. Bring to a boil and simmer 20 minutes. Use tamari to taste. Add noodles and bring to a boil; then take off heat.

Rice Tea:

Sick children sometimes have no appetite. Rice tea is good nourishment when this happens.

Roast 1 cup rice until brown. Add rice to 10 cups water and cook 30 minutes. Strain and give liquid to child. If your baby has a yang condition and doesn't like rice tea, give him barley or pearl barley tea.

Charcoal medicines

Charcoal medicines are very strong. To charcoal umeboshi, kombu or top of eggplant (for dentie), use an unglazed ceramic pot with a tight-fitting lid. Fill to ⅓ capacity with food to be charcoaled. Seal the lid with bread dough to make it air tight. Bake in oven with high flame. When it starts to smoke, open oven and reduce flame to medium. Then bake for 1 hour, remove from oven and shake. You should hear the dry scraping of charcoal; if you don't hear this, bake another 10 minutes. Let cool for 30 minutes before opening lid. Grind to a powder in a suribachi.

Other Books Available from the George Ohsawa Macrobiotic Foundation:

by George Ohsawa:
Macrobiotics: The Way of Healing
The Macrobiotic Guidebook for Living
Jack and Mitie
The Book of Judgment
The Book of Judo and Flower Arrangement
You Are All Sanpaku
Zen Macrobiotics

by Herman Aihara:
Basic Macrobiotics
Acid and Alkaline
Invitation to Health and Happiness
Learning From Salmon
Sotai Natural Exercise

by Cornellia Aihara
The First Macrobiotic Cookbook
The Dō of Cooking Cookbook
The Calendar Cookbook
Macrobiotic Kitchen Cookbook
Macrobiotic Child Care
Macrobiotic Home Remedies - Healing at Home

For a complete macrobiotic book catalog and/or Foundation membership information, please send your request to the George Ohsawa Macrobiotic Foundation, 1511 Robinson St., Oroville, CA 95965, tel. (916) 533-7702.